UNDERSTANDING ADDICTION

TAMING THE TIGER WITHIN

ILLUSTRATED

WAINO SUOJANEN, Ph.d

THERESA D. WILLIAMS FIRSTER, B.S.; A.S.

To Order copies from Author:

Address: Theresa W. Firster
917 Jordan Rd.
Dacula, GA. 30019

(678)-985-1711
email: botre7@ bellsouth.net

ISBN 1-883707-40-4

First Edition

Table of Contents

Introduction

Part I – MAD Chemicals

Part II – MAD Behaviors

Chapter Five: Mad Behaviors

Compulsive Gambling

- Case Study

Overeating

- Case Study

Workaholism

- Case Study

Sexaholism

- Case Study

PART III – Transformation

Chapter Six: Transformation

Chapter Seven: Values

Chapter Eight: Beliefs

Chapter Nine: The Process of Change

Chapter Ten: Setting Goals and Creating Your

Future

INTRODUCTION

I am amazed at the lack of knowledge and the misconception people have concerning addiction. In my own family, a daughter-in-law who is a nurse told me, "We don't' need to intervene with Dad's drinking; all he needs is more attention and love from his family." I was appalled at the lack of knowledge from an individual who supposedly understood physiology and medicine. It took a physical crisis before the family (and Dad) admitted there was a problem.

There seems to be a blind spot in our society that refuses to see the insidiousness of alcohol and drugs. It is almost sacrilegious to infer that someone "drinks" too much. In some elements of society it is almost a rite of passage into adulthood. It's a sign of intestinal fortitude and strength to brag about how drunk you got the night before.

For family and friends of the drunk, it becomes a puzzle. "How do we deal with this? Can't he see what he's doing to himself and others?" The answer is no, he feels he doesn't have a problem, you do! Addiction is a disease that tells you, you don't have it.

Addiction is insidious. It eventually affects every aspect of one's life until life itself becomes unmanageable. Hopefully, this book will offer the reader a better understanding of chemical addiction and addictive behavior, as well as offering guidelines to more successful living.

Until recently, culture was considered the major factor in determining a person's behavior. But current studies show that some behaviors may be genetically programmed; that biology is a determining factor in the destiny of human animal life. Man follows what he physically feels, rather than what he intellectually knows is best. In other words, man not only relates to life through his cultural learning but often responds from the basic instincts of the animal within.

This sheds new light on why so many "techniques of change" fail. How you react to life biologically and chemically has been relatively ignored as a contributing factor to one's irresponsible behavior. Changing is not just a matter of rationally deciding that "I am going to stop this behavior," but recognizing all aspects of the problem: the emotional, intellectual and the physical.

Throughout this book we will attempt to clarify for the reader why the addict uses MAD (Mind-Altering-Drugs) chemicals, and MAD (Maladaptive-Addictive-Disorder) behaviors and why the emotions, the intellect, and physical chemistry must be considered in order to make a lasting change in the addict's lifestyle.

We use the acronym, ACORN, (addictive, compulsive, obsessive, really nutty person) to describe irresponsible behavior, and the OAK (Open, Adaptable,

Knowledgeable person) to describe responsible behavior.

Alcoholism is used as the basic model of a MAD chemical, mainly because alcohol is by far the most commonly used, abused, and addictive chemical in the western world. We also present case studies of MAD behavior such as gambling, overeating, workaholism, sexaholism to show the relationship between addictive drugs and addictive behaviors.

ACKNOWLEDGEMENTS

Each individual is unique. What works for one person may not work for another. We have tapped many resources to give the reader a choice of methods to find one that works for them. In the process we have tried to give credit where credit is due. If we have failed to do so, it is not by intent, but by the fact that it is hard to delineate where our own experience and philosophy overlaps with others. We want to fully acknowledge the numerous resources that helped us put together a book that may be of help to families and individuals dealing with the painful problem of addiction.

Awaken The Giant Within. Tony Robbins

Relaxation and Stress Reduction Work Book. Davis, MacKay and Eshelman

A Guide to Rational Living. Albert Ellis

Values Clarification. Louis & Raths

Illusions. Richard Bach

Cover Design. Dean Funk

PART I

MAD CHEMICALS

EMOTIONAL

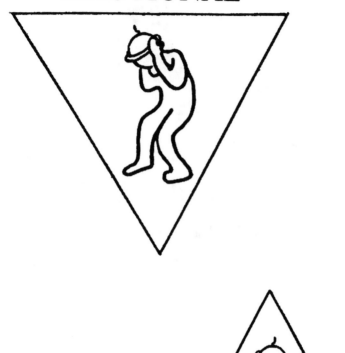

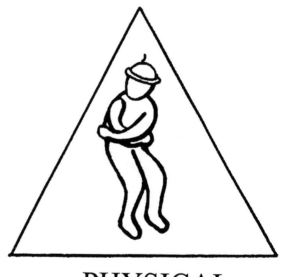

PHYSICAL

ADDICTION

CHAPTER ONE

UNDERSTANDING ADDICTION

"WHILE ADDICTION ITSELF CAN TAKE MANY FORMS, THERE ARE ONLY TWO KINDS OF ADDICTION: PHYSICAL ADDICTION THAT IS CONTROLLED BY THE BODY, AND EMOTIONAL ADDICTION, WHICH IS CONTROLLED BY THE MIND."

What is addiction? The dictionary defines it as "to devote or surrender (oneself) to something habitually or obsessively. To cause (one) to become physiologically dependent upon a drug." In other words, addiction is a dependence on something outside yourself that becomes so excessive it noticeably interferes with your physical health and your ability to relate realistically with others.

Do you know someone who:

- Has a problem with overeating?

- Takes drugs to get up in the morning and to go to sleep at night?

- Needs a drink to unwind in the evening?

- Is so obsessed with gambling that he/she has lost everything?

- Works 80-hour weeks?

- Has uncontrollable sexual urges?

If so, this book offers the reader a better understanding and a new perspective on how destructive behavior and addiction:

- Affects one physically;

- Why people use MAD chemicals (Mind-Altering-Drugs);

- And MAD behaviors (Maladaptive Addictive Disorders) to cope with life;

- And what the addicted person and family needs to create a concrete practical program for change.

While addiction itself can take many forms, there are only two kinds of addiction: physical addiction, which is controlled by the body, and emotional addiction, which is controlled by the mind. Until recently, science denied any physical and emotional connection within the body. It was thought in the early days of medicine that the heart controlled behavior and the brain was simply an organ that cooled the blood. But, scientists today have a better understanding of how the mind and body work together to create the whole.

Though chemicals control both physical and psychological addictions, they affect different parts of the brain.

Understanding how the brain controls these chemicals is an important aspect of this book. To understand how this works let's look more closely at how the brain works.

CHAPTER TWO

ADDICTION AND THE BRAIN

> 'EACH PART OF THE BRAIN IS IN CHARGE OF DIFFERENT BEHAVIORS. THE LEFT NEW BRAIN ASKS 'WHAT ARE THE FACTS?' THE RIGHT NEW BRAIN ASKS 'WHAT ARE THE SOLUTIONS?' AND THE OLD BRAIN ASKS 'HOW DOES IT FEEL?''

There are three main parts to the brain. The New or human brain is divided into two sections – the *Left New Brain* (LNB) and the *Right New Brain* (RNB). The *Visceral Brain* (VB) or Old Brain is located around the brain stem and contains the pleasure and pain areas of the body ... all three working together create what is called the Integrative Mind, or what we also refer to as the Tri-une Brain.

LEFT

WHY?

HOW?

NOW!

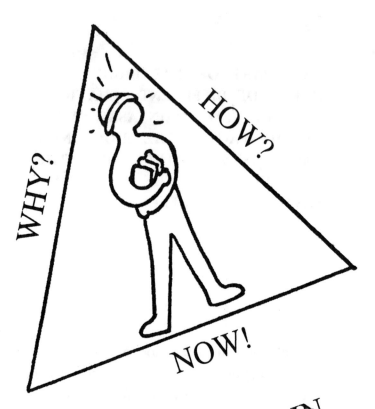

NEW BRAIN

Each part of the brain is in charge of different behaviors.

The *Left New Brain* is:

> Analytical
>
> Quantitative
>
> Intellectual
>
> Verbal
>
> Rational

When you use words, do arithmetic and think logically and rationally, you are using the LNB. The person who functions mainly from the left brain is the type of individual who always walks, moves and eats rapidly; measures everything in numbers; hurries more and more as time passes; very much a perfectionist; everything is either black or white and she/he usually has a narrow focus of beliefs. Every project is a command performance; his co-workers respect him for his ability to get things done, but also curse him because he demands perfection from them also and doesn't hesitate to point out their character defects when necessary.

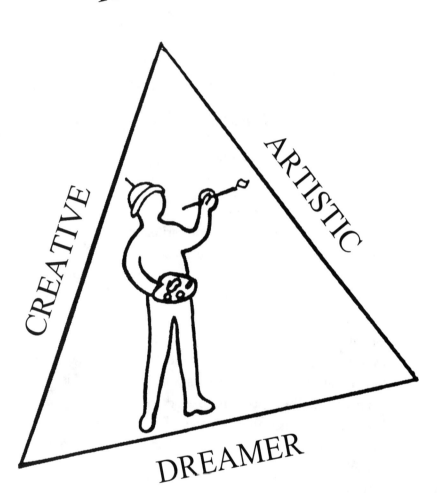

RIGHT

ARTISTIC

CREATIVE

DREAMER

NEW BRAIN

The LNB individual can be called a sense-feel-think person and tends to be very dogmatic and methodical, seldom bending a rule. Everything must be done by the book. Nearly all testing done in schools focuses on the functioning of the LNB because it can be measured. These tests almost totally ignore the fact that the creative right brain and the feeling Old Brain are very important to the complete functioning of the individual.

The *Right New Brain* is quite different in its functions. It governs:

Creativity

Artistic skills

Synthesizing

Spatial design

The individual who functions predominantly from the Right Brain is often an artist or craftsman. Absent is the logic and balance of the Left Brain. RNB's tend to daydream and live in a world filled with fantasies. They are also initiators of new and creative ideas but can't be bothered with the details of how to get things done. The person with a dominant Right Brain prefers less structure.

15

VISCERAL

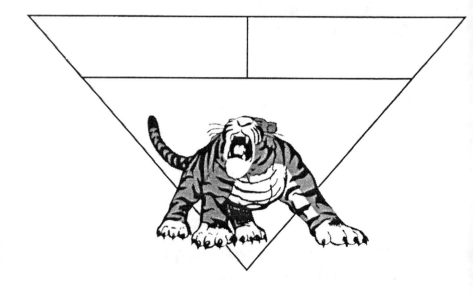

BRAIN

RNB's are called sense-feel-create people because they tend to build dreams, philosophize, and refuse to be pinned down to one focus.

The *Visceral Brain*, or what is sometimes referred to as the "Old Brain" controls the animal drives of man as well as his motivational and emotional behavior. The old brain and the newer higher brains in humans are always warring for control. During times of stress, the old brain nearly always wins. With its swift chemical responses, the old brain checks out the situation and reacts according to how it "feels."

In times of threat or danger, the "Old Brain" shifts into automatic. This response is called the Fight or Flight response (FFR) and is stimulated as the hypothalamus (located in the visceral brain) acts chemically on the adrenal glands. They in turn produce the chemical epinephrine (adrenaline) which acts on the cells throughout the body to prepare you physically to fight or run; blood pressure rises, the heart beats faster and the muscles become tense. This instinctive, automatic response continues until the danger is past.

The incredible power of this response is demonstrated in crisis situations by giving individuals strength and abilities otherwise thought impossible. Like the one hundred-pound pianist who was able to more her 2,000-pound grand piano to save it from being destroyed in a fire, or the mother who lifted a 3,000-pound car to save the life of her child. The survival instincts of the old brain react instinctively to protect the body from immediate danger.

When the old brain takes over, control is passed from the new brain, the thinking, "human" part of the brain, to the old brain, the instinctive "animal" part of the brain. It is at this point that chemistry determines how you behave. The rational, creative mind is lost to the basic instincts of animal survival.

The VB individual is a sense-feel-do person and constantly seeks pleasure and instant gratification. She sees what she wants, feels good about wanting it, and wants it NOW!

The Visceral Brain consists of the Hind-Brain (HB), the Mid-Brain (MB), and the part of the forebrain known as the Limbic region. Limbic, which is derived from the work Limbo, means the edge or border. Limbo is defined as a place of restraint or confinement; it also means a region on the border of hell. When the addict creates the imbalance of chemicals in his brain, he creates his own limbo. When a recovering addict says, "Alcohol gave me wings to fly ... and then it took away the sky," it is an attempt to describe the torment and pain of a self-imposed limit with its initial sense of power and freedom and the inevitable tailspin back to reality.

In a crisis, when time is of the essence, the old brain becomes the decision-maker. It acts on instinct and feelings and makes decisions based on the five senses alone.

While the old brain controls the five senses, the two new brains working together as a unit control reality. This balance creates decisions based on emotional, intellectual and physical considerations.

When an individual is out of balance, that is, reacting to life from a purely emotional state, he is

falling back on the old brain, basing his behavior on instinctual feelings without the balance of reason and logic, reverting to the "animal" within. We call this type of individual an ACORN, an **A**ddictive, **C**ompulsive, **O**bsessive, **R**eally **N**utty person who is hooked on MAD behaviors or MAD chemicals or often both.

An OAK on the other hand is someone who is **O**pen, **A**daptable, and **K**nowledgeable and approaches life with an optimistic outlook. He sees life as a gift to be cherished, a gift that must be developed through a balanced lifestyle.

OAK

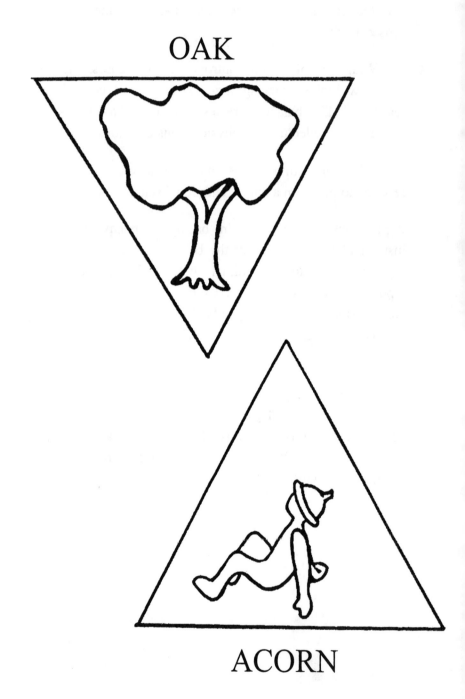

ACORN

CHAPTER THREE

THE ACORN AND THE OAK

How well you manage your life depends on your knowledge, attitudes, and behavior. Knowledge changes attitudes, attitudes affect behavior, and how you behave makes you perform either as an ACORN or an OAK.

Nature's Acorn is created with a genetic program that gives it the potential of becoming an Oak, but many fall on fallow ground. The human ACORN is also born with the potential to soar and grow, but without proper nourishment and understanding, that potential can languish unnoticed and unfulfilled. With a sense of hopelessness and failure, many ACORNS turn to drugs, alcohol, gambling, overeating, sex and working too hard just to make life bearable.

The ACORN relies on a MAD chemical or MAD behavior to reduce anxiety and to make life bearable. Sooner or later he becomes dependent on the chemical and/or behavior and, when this occurs, he crosses the invisible line to addiction. The ACORN seeks "better

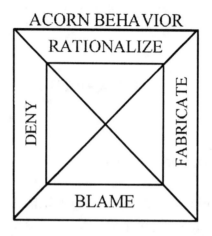

ACORN BEHAVIOR

RATIONALIZE

DENY

FABRICATE

BLAME

IRRESPONSIBLE BEHAVIOR

The behavior of a person addicted to a MAD chemical or to a MAD behavior or any combination of the two, will deny, rationalize, blame, and fabricate when confronted by a situation which s/he cannot control.

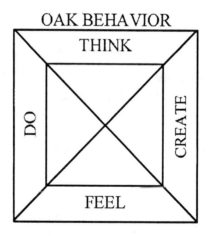

OAK BEHAVIOR

THINK

DO

CREATE

FEEL

RESPONSIBLE BEHAVIOR

The OAK is responsible for everything that she does, thinks, feels, or creates. A responsible human being is one who operates by the value which states, "If I'm not the problem, there is no solution."

things for better living through biochemistry" or "pours high voltage chemicals into low voltage situations." He cannot face life without his MAD chemicals or MAD behavior and uses them as crutches to limp through life. These crutches permit him to simply exist – as opposed to living.

The chemicals that the addict uses are called sensual drugs because they "turn-on" the pleasure areas of the brain. Regular use of these drugs creates dependency. Once the body becomes dependent on a chemical that is administered externally, it ceases to produce those chemicals internally. When those chemicals are withdrawn, it takes the brain a long time to return to its natural level. The body goes into temporary shock while the brain attempts to adjust. Withdrawal from a Mind-Altering Drug or chemical can be life threatening. All systems of the body have become dependent on it and in its absence, the ACORN will shake and hallucinate and even go into convulsions.

As an example: Tom was suffering from alcohol withdrawal when his friends brought him into the emergency room of the hospital. In spite of the measures taken to save his life, Tom died. Apparently, he had gone into withdrawal at an Alcoholics Anonymous meeting and well meaning friends had been trying to help by feeding him orange juice. They thought the sugar in the juice would be enough to keep his system functioning. Sugar couldn't replace the chemicals that his brain and body desperately needed to find balance. If detoxification had been performed earlier under medical supervision, the patient might have survived. (Detoxification is the process of slowly withdrawing an individual from a drug by replacing it with a medical drug or by a gradual weaning from the drug itself. This allows the body to stabilize.)

To the ACORN, an addictive behavior or addictive chemical initially provides immediate pleasure. He has difficulty seeing what the future can hold for him and focuses on short-term pleasures in an attempt to create joy or satisfaction in his life.

CHAPTER FOUR

ALCOHOLISM

THE ALCOHOLIC

"THE UNIVERSAL QUESTION IS 'WHY DON'T THEY SEE WHAT'S HAPPENING TO THEM?' THE ANSWER IS, THEY CAN'T. ADDICTION IS A DISEASE THAT TELLS YOU, YOU DON'T HAVE IT."

Alcoholism is a disease. Unchecked it is 100% fatal. The recovering alcoholic learns to live with his disease; he does not overcome it. It cannot be cured; it can only be arrested. With each binge, the alcoholic finds himself right where he left off and the disease continues to destroy him.

As the addiction/disease progresses, the individual loses self-esteem, becomes more deluded, less aware of his own behavior and eventually loses touch with his emotions entirely. The universal question is "why don't they see what's happening to them?" The answer is, they can't. Addiction is a disease that tells you, you don't have it.

William lived with his disease for over twenty-five years. He came from a family with a domineering, alcoholic father and a whining mother. As the only son, he was expected to take over his father's construction business, which he detested, with his mother's admonition "it will destroy him if you don't." Out of guilt and frustration, William did as he was told and began to emulate his father not only in the construction business but also as a practicing alcoholic.

Alcohol slowly erodes every area of the alcoholic's life … as Williams says, "My first marriage was a disaster. My wife attempted suicide and had spells of deep depression. She spent many years in an institution for the mentally ill. When she was eventually well enough to be released, she asked for a divorce. Unfortunately, at a time when she was about to begin a new life, she was killed in an airplane crash.

"My second wife, a childhood friend, struggled with me through the worst years of my drinking. I found alcohol to be the cheapest means of escaping from reality. If there is any motive for drinking, it is this desire to escape from intolerable situations.

"The turning point came for me when my wife decided she wanted a temporary separation. My memories of the separation are vague; I was in an alcoholic stupor most of the time. When she finally called to say she would be back the next day, I went to the store, bought a quarter of whiskey and drank far into the night. In the morning, I showered and dressed meticulously, finished off the rest of the whiskey and waited. As she walked into the sunroom where I was sitting, I stood up, stretched myself tall and unceremoniously fell flat on my face.

"When I woke up the next morning I was surprised to find that I wasn't shaking. I usually needed that first shot in the morning to calm me, but for some reason this morning I was fine. Instead of reaching for a drink, I reached for the phone and called my doctor and said, I need help, meet me at the hospital. I began my road back to reality with medical help and the support of Alcoholics Anonymous."

When the ACORN has become hooked, his brain shouts "more-more." His addiction becomes a "cup" around him and he begins to create elaborate defenses to protect his habit. As the disease progresses, these defenses become more and more rigid and begin to invade his very lifestyle. He finds it difficult to adapt to change, particularly unexpected change. This kind of ACORN becomes an almost impossible "nut" to crack.

Jim was another "tough nut." He began drinking at the early age of twelve by sneaking drinks from the Church's supply of communion wine. For Jim, this was the beginning of forty years of alcoholism.

Jim came from a family of alcoholics. As a young boy he secretly sipped from his father's cache of liquor, replacing it with water. At twenty-six Jim was a full-blown alcoholic. In college, he continued his drinking, using excuses such as his shyness with people and especially with women. It was during this time his doctor began giving him Valium and Darvon (minor tranquilizers) for a back problem. Jim became cross-addicted; not only addicted to alcohol, but to prescription drugs as well.

Jim states, "As with many alcoholics, I thought a geographic move would cure my problem. It didn't, it just followed me wherever I went. I tried every excuse to keep from admitting that I had a problem.

"It was on a business trip to New Orleans that I realized I desperately needed to do something; I couldn't go on the way I had been. There was no great vision, no great moment of truth. I just knew I needed help. My wife and I took a plane home and I signed myself into the hospital. In accepting the fact that I am an alcoholic, I eventually learned that I had to give up everything related to drinking ... friends, hobbies, places. I had to restructure my life. Working with Alcoholics Anonymous, I began to build a workable schedule to fill the void of drinking, and was able to create a more constructive lifestyle for myself."

Even though Jim stated that there was no great vision, no great moment of truth when he decided to seek help, studies have shown that this decision is usually reached after many crises have occurred as a result of the disease. The deterioration of their lives forces the individual to recognize the problem.

The ego strength of the alcoholic is almost nonexistent. Their defenses are rigid and they become totally unaware of their actions. When an addict hits bottom and finally accepts that he is powerless over the addiction, he has taken the first step. This is the beginning of his program of change. Change can only be achieved by complete surrender; which means recognizing that he must let go of old habits and beliefs. There must be a personality change as well as a releasing of the negative addiction.

Along with constructing a new lifestyle, the alcoholic or drug addict must be cautious of prescription drugs and over-the-counter drugs because both of these can be very deadly.

A case in point was Bob, a recovering alcoholic. His doctor prescribed antihistamines for his allergy. The medication had the same effect on him as alcohol. Once he came off the antihistamines, he experienced the same terrible torture of withdrawal that he had with alcohol. He was fortunate that he was active in the AA program and was able, with help, to get back into his program of recovery.

Betty, also a recovering alcoholic, was not so fortunate. She went to the drugstore and bought a cough medicine that stated it contained no alcohol. What she didn't know was that it did contain an artificial opiate. The reaction to the opiate caused her to slip back into her old drinking habits. She died in an automobile accident two weeks later.

The individual must be responsible and exercise caution when taking drugs and medication since doctors are not always aware of the addictive properties of prescriptions and over-the-counter drugs. It is almost impossible for the medical profession to keep up with the proliferation of drugs on the market. Self-help programs such as Alcoholics Anonymous and Narcotics Anonymous can be of much more help than professionals who have not experienced life in the pits of polydrug addiction.

Alcohol, along with other drugs, is cunning, baffling, and powerful. The resulting disease involves the individual at many levels: physically, mentally, emotionally, and spiritually. The progress of the disease can be halted and the individual can recover but the alcoholic or drug addict is never cured. Once you become hooked, you live in a world which can neither be imagined nor understood by those who have not lived in that world. Whenever anyone attempts to help an addict, they must remember that addiction is like a third person in a relationship. The first person is the addict; the second person is the helper; and the third is the addiction. One of the reasons AA succeeds where professional therapists fail is that self-help group members know their "third-party." They have lived with it for extended periods of time. No one can understand an addict as well as another addict.

The dedicated ACORN loses touch with reality, because the mixed-up chemicals in his brain give him a distorted view of life. This distortion is also created with MAD behaviors. Whenever we create a behavior pattern that is so excessive it noticeably interferes with our physical health, or intellectual and spiritual development, it becomes impossible for us to relate and interact with others on a realistic basis. Overeaters, workaholics, smokers, gamblers, and sexaholics, refuse to recognize their addiction.

PART II

MAD BEHAVIORS

CHAPTER FIVE

MAD BEHAVIORS

> "THE VERY SAME CHEMICALS THAT CREATE THE HIGH FOR THE ALCOHOLIC AND DRUG USER ARE 'NATURALLY' CREATED FOR THE GAMBLER AND OVEREATER, THE WORKAHOLIC AND THE SEXAHOLIC."

Why does the addict or ACORN behave in such a destructive manner? The reasons are many and complex, but the process by which people become dependent on chemicals is the same as for those who become hooked on negative behaviors. Chemical addiction and emotional addiction are closely related. The very same chemicals that create the high for the alcoholic and drug user are "naturally" created for the gambler and overeater, the workaholic and the sexaholic. The rush or high of natural adrenaline is as potent for them as an externally administered chemical. The endorphins, our natural painkillers, have been compared to morphine. They not only have the ability to blunt pain, but also produce a peculiar state of indifference and emotional detachment from the experience of suffering.

As you will see, MAD behavior, can stimulate the brain to produce that state of bliss which allows the addict to escape ... albeit temporarily, from his problem or state of boredom.

THE GAMBLER

Mike escaped his boredom through gambling. At 23, he was one of the youngest members of Gamblers Anonymous when he attended his first meeting in 1958. At that time, gambling was barely recognized as an addiction.

Mike knew by the age of thirteen that he was a compulsive gambler. It began innocently enough with a baseball flipping contest. He remembers it so vividly, because it was the first time he sensed that rush of adrenaline, that quickening of the pulse and feeling of exhilaration that came with winning or losing.

Since Mike came from the Country Club set, his gambling wasn't from lack of the good life. The end goal wasn't really what he was after. Rather, it was his compulsion and need for that rush or high of adrenaline – from the activity itself. It was only when Mike was on the verge of being caught for a serious burglary with the fear of prison hanging over his head that he stopped to take a look at his life. He didn't like what he saw. All the spiritual principles that he believed in had broken down. He was no longer the person he wanted to be. It was then that he went to his first Gamblers Anonymous (GA) meeting with the resolve and decision to change his life.

Mike was hooked on the high of gambling. Just as the alcoholic experiences withdrawal, Mike also went through a form of withdrawal with long periods of sleeplessness, nervousness, loss of appetite and a general lack of concern for his physical needs. Because he relied so heavily on his MAD behavior – the gambling – to create excitement in his life, he now had to find other ways to create more positive and realistic ways of meeting life on its own terms.

When life seems to be handing us a poor hand, we try to ease the pain and frustration through other means. Too often we look for the quick fix, the jury rig, and instant rewards. When we don't get them we go back to MAD chemicals and MAD behavior.

THE OVEREATER

Another way we get our "fix" is with food. Beverly was an overeater. She didn't begin to have a problem until after she was settled into married life. She loved cooking for her family and as her family grew, so did Beverly. With each pregnancy, she found herself gaining first five, then ten, then twenty pounds, until with the birth of her third child she weighed over 180 pounds.

Although Beverly spent years trying one diet after another, she was never able to keep her weight down. The process of her dieting created chaos in her life. Her temperament flowed like the waves of the ocean, high one moment and deeply depressed the next. She finally realized and accepted that she was addicted. She was never far from that which she loved the most – food. To be closer to the kitchen, Beverly would sit on the sofa waiting for her last meal to digest, thinking about what she was going to eat next. Just thinking about more food made her euphoric. While she recognized that there was something very sick about what she was doing, she knew of no way to control it.

Beverly did eventually go into therapy. It helped her to understand her behavior, but it didn't help to control it. As she states, "I feel one of the weaknesses of therapy was that I was given permission to pamper myself, which is what I was already doing. Eventually I joined Overeaters Anonymous (OA)." OA is a fellowship for people with an overeating addiction who share their experiences, strength, and hope to solve their common problem. In OA Beverly learned she could change her life; that compulsive overeating, like alcoholism, was a disease. Only when the disease is under control can you turn your attention to other areas of your life.

Beverly adds, "Although the support of the OA groups is important, I have to realize that if I am not the problem, there is no solution. Only I am responsible for my behavior. If someone is not there to help me at a time when I need it, I must be the one who chooses not to eat or go on that binge. Maintaining my equilibrium is my responsibility not somebody else's.

"More than the support of the group members, I found the spirituality of the program has helped me to live on a higher level. In the past, I was always filled with anxiety, but having accepted that there is a higher power helping me, I feel as if I'm not alone. I now have a constant source of help in controlling my MAD behavior. I have become more tolerant of myself and others as a result of my program."

Accepting responsibility and a change in attitude is part of the foundation of recovery. The compulsive overeater must accept that he or she is powerless over the disease and reach out for the support needed to cope with the problem.

Although the gambler and the overeater may consider themselves unique in their problems, the same thread runs through the lives of the workaholic and the sexaholic. All four are ACORNS. The therapy that works for one will work for all. In the ACORN, the body, the mind, and the spirit are held captive by a chemical jailer whether it is those bought in the store or on the street, or those produced by the brain and the body of the ACORN. MAD chemicals and MAD behaviors are roads to oblivion.

THE WORKAHOLIC

Dan's escape was work. His life consisted of study, work and family. He had set up such a rigorous schedule for himself that it left little time for fun. Dan attempted to maintain a career, work on a Master's degree and find time for his family. Through the years this juggling act became more and more difficult to maintain. As Dan states, "I can't even let myself enjoy taking a shower anymore. I keep thinking of the things I should be doing instead. I pushed my body to the pure limits of survival, sacrificing rest to balance other aspects of my life. Even when I was aware that I was reaching my limit, the "High" I received from completing a project successfully just reinforced my wanting more. If I didn't have another project ready to go, I would experience a period of what I recognized as withdrawal symptoms: insomnia and nervousness that left me in a cold sweat and my temper on edge. I finally accepted that workaholism is an addiction, and that I was addicted. I was powerless over my MAD behavior and my life had become unmanageable.

In common with the alcoholic or drug addict, the workaholic fails to see his problem until he is pushed to extremes. It is only when he is forced to face reality does he make that choice to change his life. Only he can make that decision.

THE SEXAHOLIC

Lisa thought she had a unique problem. She was a sexaholic. It is not commonly accepted that sex can be an addiction, but it is proven to be just as destructive as other forms of addiction. As Lisa relates, "It all started four years ago in London. I was footloose and fancy free, and honestly believed that I didn't need anybody or anything. I treated what few interpersonal relationships I had like treasure from some pirated ship. What was mine was whatever I could beg, borrow or steal, or worse yet plunder (affairs, usually someone else's husband). Men were the reward for a day or night's work. The more I worked, the more I wanted. Little did I realize that I had become addicted. It was not to drugs, alcohol or work. It was the social no-no, a Biblical "God'll getcha," it was sex. Like many addicts, I always said I could swear off the stuff anytime. Unfortunately, it wasn't that easy. I was well into those biological cravings that every addict gets when he or she has developed an unusually high tolerance level for a drug, or whatever. The plundering became more frequent, and the specific events, names, faces, and facts became more and more blurred. It wasn't unusual for me not to remember or even be concerned about the name or face of the person I had just been with. Finally, like so many addicts, I hit bottom. I was lucky enough not to hit absolute rock bottom, but came close enough to realize that things had gotten terribly out of hand. I finally decided that I could only maintain one life successfully. My other life was quite unknown to my family and few friends. In looking back, I realized that although my affairs were many, I had never attempted to maintain a lasting relationship. I didn't even know how to start a relationship with some degree of permanency. I read somewhere that to have a friend you have to be a friend. In Sexaholics Anonymous (SA), I have learned to be my own best friend before I can actually reach out and be a friend to another.

"Learning to be my own best friend was perhaps one of the most difficult experiences of my life. No matter what I said to me, I always knew the truth. I had to take responsibility for my actions, who I was and what I had done to myself. I had to learn to love me. I also discovered that I could not run away from myself. Learning to accept was a problem. I had to learn to accept without judging and without condition. It was at this point I began to rebuild my life."

Moving from the slavery of the ACORN to the independence of the OAK can be highly traumatic. Self-help groups call this process "no pain-no gain." Whenever you choose a different path you must give up the old path. It is not possible to keep one foot on each and progress. You must change your playgrounds and your playmates. It takes courage and willingness to transform your life from an ACORN to an OAK.

42

PART III

TRANSFORMATION

CHAPTER SIX

TRANSFORMATION FROM ACORN TO OAK

"INWARD CHANGE DEMANDS A DRASTIC ALTERATION IN YOUR THOUGHT PATTERNS."

Transformation from ACORN to OAK requires three things:

1. Recognizing that your ACORN behavior is causing the problem.

2. A willingness to be responsible for your actions.

3. A realization that change is continuous; life is a journey not a destination.

These are the main elements necessary to begin designing a program that will transform your life. By recognizing that "you" are the problem, it follows that "you" are the solution. Your negative behaviors create the negative consequences of those behaviors. New results demand new behaviors.

Change comes from within. When you use chemicals or negative behaviors to stimulate the pleasure areas of the brain, your acting on the belief that pleasure can only come from without. Inward change demands a drastic alteration in your thought patterns. You change your thought patterns and create balance in your life by examining your values and beliefs.

A balanced life requires that all three parts of the brain work together as a whole:

The Left New Brain – the analytical side

asks: "What are the Facts?"

The Right New Brain – the creative part

asks: "What are the solutions?"

The Visceral Brain – the emotional side

asks: "How does it feel?"

In most instances, people initially make decisions based largely at the feeling level of the brain. They *react* from a set of values and beliefs developed in childhood without testing their validity from an adult point of view. Our choices are often made based on these infantile emotions.

The willingness to create and make new choices based on a more mature understanding takes courage. Richard Bach expresses it beautifully in his book, Illusions. He tells of a village of creatures that lived along the bottom a great crystal river, each creature clung tightly to twigs and rocks on the river bottom. "For clinging was their way of life and resisting the current what each had learned from birth. But one of the creatures, out of boredom, let go of his rock and was tumbled and smashed by the current, yet in time the current lifted him free from the bottom and he was bruised and hurt no more."

When you first begin to take responsibility for your life, when you start thinking for yourself, you run into opposition. By going against the status quo, you are tumbled and dashed against the rocks of "tradition," "society," or the "right" way to do things. But once you have tested it and are no longer afraid to let go and be yourself, others have less power over you to "make" you hurt.

Letting go of "other's" values places the responsibility of making choices squarely on your shoulders. A sometimes frightening prospect! According to psychological studies, by the time you reach seven years old, your brain is pretty well imprinted with the values and beliefs of others. We are all a blend of our parents, peers, teachers, television, advertisers, and society as a whole.

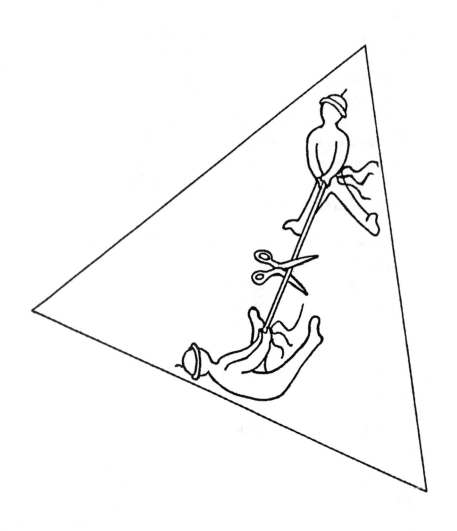

The brain of a child is like a sponge, absorbing everything around him in an attempt to make some sense out of the world. In this process, his experience will build his perception of the world. If as a child your father beat you consistently, the message your brain received was that men inflict pain and are to be feared. It will take a lot of understanding and awareness as an adult to change that perception. The stronger the emotion, the stronger the imprint left on the brain.

In fact, it has been shown in recent studies, that there is an actual physical connection made in the brain when you do something for the first time. With each repetition it increases the tensile strength of this connection. It soon becomes an automatic pathway to that feeling or behavior when a similar situation arises. When that connection is triggered, your brain automatically pulls from the strongest pathways surrounding similar experiences in an effort to resolve and understand the current situation. This explains why it is so difficult to break old habits. It is not just a matter of thinking your way out of behavior, but literally cutting the *physical* link to the past.

Having someone else set your values makes life comfortable. The guidelines are set. But if your life isn't working it's time to question whether those values and beliefs from the past are still valid.

Clarifying and re-creating your values gives you a map for the future. It helps define what is important to you in life and a guideline that lets you know if you are on the right road.

By accepting responsibility for your actions, you have the power to change. By taking each day at a time, change becomes more manageable. Being less fearful and willing to let go of old values and beliefs, you can begin to build a new foundation.

The process of building a new foundation involves becoming aware of your actions and your thoughts and how they contribute to your present problems. Getting to know yourself is not an easy task because of:

HABITS: You do things routinely, without thinking about them.

TRAINING: You look to other authority figures to give you a sense of worth – your rightness or wrongness.

HOPING: Hoping someone or something out there will make things right for you.

JUDGING: You deny your feelings through the process of judging (shoulds, shouldn'ts, I shouldn't be angry, etc.)

Changing values and beliefs can be very threatening as the following situation illustrates:

During a family retreat workshop, the instructor was discussing values when the minister jumped to his feet, obviously agitated and demanded to know what was wrong with his father's values. If they were good enough for his father, they were good enough for him.

The instructor tried to calm the minister by explaining that it is perfectly acceptable to agree with your parents values if you have given them due thought and examination and then ... accepted them as your own.

What are values? Values are labels you give to whatever is important in your life. They have different levels of importance, depending on how strongly you feel about them. Values regulate, discipline and shape your life, pointing you in the direction of either success or failure.

CHAPTER SEVEN

VALUES

> "Your values and beliefs can fairly
>
> Well predict your level of future
>
> Success or failure."
>
> Tony Robbins"

Changing your values changes the priorities of your life, the way you evaluate things, the way you behave and your ultimate future. An example of a value is not: "owning a big car, a big house and having lots of money." What you *value* is the *feeling* you get from having a big car, a big house and lots of money, a feeling of success and accomplishment.

The screen of your life experiences filters the way you perceive life. If you were taught values of distrust, intolerance, hatred and insecurity, the choices you make in life will be based on these negative values. If you

POSITIVE ATTITUDES

ATTITUDE	PERSONALITY	RESULTS
UNDERSTANDING	ENTHUSIASTIC	SUCCESS
ANTICIPATION	DECISIVE	RECOGNITION
EXPECTATION	COURAGEOUS	SECURITY
CONFIDENCE	OPTIMISTIC	ENERGY
PATIENCE	CHEERFUL	ACHIEVEMENT
HUMILITY	CONSIDERATE	HAPPINESS
BELIEF	FRIENDLY	GROWTH
	COURTEOUS	ADVENTURE
	SINCERE	HEALTH
	WARM	FRIENDSHIP
	RELAXED	LOVE

NEGATIVE ATTITUDES

ATTITUDE	PERSONALITY	RESULTS
ENVY	INCONSIDERATE	WORRY
GREED	PESSIMISTIC	TENSION
ANGER	CRUEL	DESPONDENCY
CONCEIT	WEAK	FRUSTRATION
CYNICISM	COLD	JOB WEARINESS
SELF-PITY	RUDE	UNHAPPINESS
SUSPICION	SOUR	FAILURE
INDECISION	DRAB	SICKNESS
CRITICISM	IRRITABLE	POVERTY
INFERIORITY	UNDETERMINED	LONELINESS

[Chart No. 1]

have been taught positive values such as integrity, honesty, love and service, your attitude and choices will reflect these values. "Your values and beliefs can fairly well predict your level of future success or failure." (Tony Robbins, Awaken the Giant Within). Someone who believes in him/herself and has a fairly positive outlook on life will persist in the face of obstacles because he ultimately believes in success. The person who lacks confidence is always looking for the worst to happen and subconsciously doesn't believe she can have it anyway. If you don't believe it's possible, why even try?

Chart No. [1] shows how a positive or negative attitude will affect your personality. Your attitudes and personality reflect your values and beliefs, which in turn determine behavior.

Positive values give stability and consistency to your life. Unfortunately this same consistency can create problems. Example: If one of your values is "to be nice to people at all costs" and you become angry with a friend, your value will get in the way of your expressing that anger. The stronger the value, the more difficult it becomes to accept and express the feelings that conflict with that value. Your value system acts like a filter that directs and guides the way you respond to life.

Begin by clarifying your own values. What do you want from life? What is important to you? A method used successfully by others was developed by co-authors Louis and Rath in their book <u>Values Clarification.</u> The authors offer you criteria to judge each value. They are as follows:

1. **PRIZING AND CHERISHING**

   Are you proud of your position?

2. **PUBLICLY AFFIRMING**, when appropriate.

   Are you willing to stand up for what you believe?

3. **CHOOSING FROM ALTERNATIVES**

   Did you choose them after due consideration?

4. **CHOOSING AFTER CONSIDERATION OF THE CONSEQUENCES**

   Did you choose after careful consideration?

5. **CHOOSING FREELY**

   Have you chosen your position freely with no coercion or guilt involved?

6. **ACTING**

   Have you acted on or done anything about your beliefs?

7. **ACTING WITH A PATTERN** or consistency on this issue.

Is it really a part of you?

Following is a list that will give you a clearer idea of what a value is. As an exercise, choose five most important values and then put them in the order of importance. You should be able to give an explanation in support of your belief.

PERSONAL VALUES

1. All people regardless of race, sex, or creed should be treated equally.

2. Democracy expresses the will of the people and should, therefore, be preserved at all costs, including the interest and participation of all the people.

3. Belief in God.

4. Excesses in any form should be excluded from one's life – excesses in eating, recreation, even work are examples.

5. Regardless of the criminal or immoral behavior of others, they are human beings and should be treated with compassion, respect, and appropriate dignity.

6. One should refrain from lying, stealing or cheating.

7. No other gods must be placed before the one you believe in.

8. Rights and feelings of others should be respected.

9. The very process of swearing is dependent on degrading verbal symbols and converting language into ugliness; it should be avoided.

10. A sound set of personal ethics and standards must be established for proper conduct and success in one's working career.

After having completed the above exercise, take the time to write out your own values. Following are some suggestions that will assist in the process:

1. Write down ten things you **LIKE TO DO.** Such as activities, jogging, swimming, reading, etc. Be aware that if you say you like swimming, but you never go swimming, chances are you don't value it enough to do anything about it.

2. List five additional changes you wish to make or achieve in your life. These can include any spiritual, physical, emotional, or social changes.

3. With each item, make a short statement that reflects some of your own values. For example: I **LIKE** swimming; the value you would derive from that is, I value a strong healthy body. **I WANT TO CHANGE** – the negative behaviors causing me problems. You value discipline and control in your life.

As you work on your list ask yourself – why do I like to do this? What is the end result I wish to achieve?

An important step in creating positive change is to overcome fear and to strengthen your own will. Know what you want and close your mind to those who would destroy the sense of peace and serenity you are seeking. Build your own sense of well being by filling your mind with thoughts of success, not thoughts of failure. When you fill your mind with negative thoughts, they become your master and your behavior will reflect those thoughts. Words used in a positive way build self-confidence and a greater belief in self.

CHAPTER EIGHT

BELIEFS

> "BELIEFS ARE RULES WE HAVE MADE UP TO MEASURE WHETHER OR NOT WE ARE LIVING UP TO OUR VALUES."
>
> TONY ROBBINS

The great philosopher William James said, "Believe that you possess significant reserves of health, energy and endurance, and your belief will create the fact."

What is a belief. It is an individual's opinion (certainty) of how life "should" be. Beliefs are rules we have made up to measure whether or not we are living up to our values. We often make up rules that are so difficult to meet that it is almost impossible for us to succeed. Since you made up the rules, all you have to do to change your life is to make up new rules.

To find out what your rules are in any situation, write down ... "What needs to happen for me to be successful in this situation." The simpler the rules, the easier it will be for you to achieve your goals.

You are limited only by what you believe, by what you consider possible or impossible. If you find yourself responding to opportunities with the statement, "I can't do that because," be aware that whatever comes after "because" is a limit you have put on yourself.

In church one Sunday, the minister told the story about a young woman he and his wife met on a trip to Hawaii. She impressed them because of her spirit and enthusiasm. She seemed to have boundless energy for all the climbing, touring, walking, dancing and general hectic pace of the trip. They didn't realize until much later that she had lost both legs from the knees down in an accident and was wearing artificial legs. She said that when the doctors amputated her legs they warned her she wouldn't be able to climb, hike or dance anymore, activities she had enjoyed before the accident. In spite of the doctors warnings, she decided to act "as if" she did have legs ... "the doctors are still trying to convince me that I can't do the things I'm doing," she said. You have to believe you can succeed before you attempt to move forward.

There are basically two kinds of beliefs. Generalized beliefs such as "life is ... or people are ... or God is" and then a set of rules by which you measure your beliefs. "For me to be successful I must make 3 million dollars a year, have a big home, 2.5 children, etc. If I make only 2 million dollars a year then I am not successful."

By believing you have unlimited resources, by taking time to understand what goes on within you both physically and mentally, you can bring yourself and those around you a serenity, understanding and love that is overflowing, unhampered by ignorance, resentment and anger.

When Mary N. started back into the business world after her divorce, she had to deal with the guilt of leaving her children with babysitters, of having to spend money on herself for work clothes, trying to find time to meet her own needs. After much pain and soul searching, she came to realize that as she became more confident, liked herself more, found her needs being met, she was able to pass this new sense of happiness on to her family and was able to be more open and loving with them.

If love, acceptance, and understanding are stifled within you, you cannot give it to another. How you think and feel inwardly will reflect outwardly and will act as a magnet to create your world around you. You are like the artist; the moment he conceives a painting in his mind, it is already created. He has only to put it on canvas. Believe you are a success and it is already so, you only have to act on it. Let go of the fear that keeps you from taking the steps from ACORN to OAK behavior.

CHAPTER NINE

THE PROCESS OF CHANGE

> "UNLESS AND UNTIL YOU MAKE A DEFINITE DECISION TO CHANGE, NOTHING WILL HAPPEN. YOU MUST HAVE A STRONG DESIRE AND COMMITMENT TO CHANGE, NOT BECAUSE SOMEONE ELSE WANTS YOU TO CHANGE, BUT BECAUSE YOU WANT IT. AND, YOU MUST BE WILLING TO TAKE ACTION."

Studies in Relapse Therapy (DiClemente and Prochaska, 1982) state that there are three stages of change, the decision and commitment to change, initial change and maintenance of change.

Until and unless you make a definite decision to change, nothing will happen. YOU must have a strong desire and commitment to change, not because someone else wants you to change, but because you want it. And, you must be willing to take action.

How do you change patterns of a lifetime? Being clear about what you do want from life is the first step in creating any change. In most instances, people make the decision to change only when their situation becomes intolerable or has become so painful that they are literally forced to change to survive.

A Canadian neurosurgeon conducted some experiments on the mind and found that when a person is forced to change a basic belief or viewpoint, the brain undergoes a series of nervous/electrical sensations equivalent to the most agonizing torture. Change creates fear and uncertainty because it threatens one's security and disrupts one's comfortable pattern of living.

Studies done by Michael Merzenich of the University of California, show that "when something happens for the first time and is accompanied by intense feelings, the brain actually creates a physical connection, a thin neural strand that allows us to reassess that emotion or behavior again in the future." He proved scientifically that the more we indulge in any pattern of behavior, the stronger the connection becomes. By replaying negative situations over and over again in our mind we literally/physically strengthen the destructive patterns. Breaking these patterns is no longer just a mental exercise but a physical challenge as well.

Therefore, the challenge is twofold: intellectual and physical. Intellectually you have clarified your values and beliefs and you now have a stronger foundation for change. Physically, the neural and emotional connections in the brain must be broken. Using a number of the techniques in this chapter can stop destructive thought and behavior patterns. According to Tony Robbins, author of <u>Awaken the Giant Within</u>, "if we interrupt the patterns for a long enough period of time, the neural connection will weaken and atrophy."

As you move forward through the process of change, fears connected with past experience arise that must be confronted before change can happen. The fear of making the wrong decision; fear of failure; fear of commitment; fear of rejection; fear of success. In other words, fear of the unknown. The fear that you will end up worse off than you are now. At least you know what to expect from your present situation. Even if it is painful. The comfort of the known seems less painful than the fear of the unknown. Your reasons and commitment to change must be strong enough to pull you through to the other side of the fear.

"To paraphrase the philosopher Nietzsche, "He who has a strong enough *why* can bear almost any *how*." "20 percent of any change is knowing how, but 80 percent is knowing why. If we gather a set of strong enough reasons to change, we can change in a minute something we've failed to change in years." (Tony Robbins, <u>Awaken the Giant Within</u>).

The following techniques can help you gain more control over your thoughts and behavior:

- FORCE FIELD ANALYSIS

- RELAXATION

- CONCENTRATION

- DEEP BREATHING

- SCRAMBLING

- THOUGHT STOPPING

- SELF-TALK

- MEDITATION

FORCE FIELD ANALYSIS:

In deciding to change a thought or behavior, make a list of the reasons for and against. What will happen if you don't change. What will happen if you do change. It will help you see more clearly what you will gain and what you will lose and what decision you need to make.

EXAMPLE:

NOT CHANGING	CHANGING BEHAVIOR
WHAT WILL IT COST ME?	WHAT WILL I GAIN?
HOW WILL I FEEL IF I DON'T CHANGE?	HOW WILL I FEEL IF I DO CHANGE?
WILL THE INITIAL CHANGE DESTROY ME?	WILL IT LEAD TO A NEW BEGINNING?

The key is to get strong enough reasons why the change should take place immediately, not someday in the future. If you don't want to change now, then you are not really willing to change, or you are still not clear about what you want.

RELAXATION

In my classes on relaxation, I found that most people are not aware of the tension they carry around with them all the time. Tension has become such a habit that when they finally do relax, they don't recognize the feeling.

A woman came up to me after one of my classes and said, "What did you do to me? I couldn't feel my body and I felt like I had lost control." She was visibly shaken and did not return to class. The process of relaxing her body was so foreign to her that she didn't understand what was happening.

Learn to discover the tension in your body. After taking a deep breath, mentally observe what happens to your body. Do the shoulders drop? Do your muscles relax or are you still holding tension in your jaw, your hands, you legs. Even while going off to sleep at night, take a deep breath and command your body to let go, and then observe where you unknowingly carry tension even when you think you are resting.

During a crisis situation, Mary used a relaxation technique she had learned in class. Just before coming out of relaxation, she was given the suggestion that by taking a deep breath she would be able to remember and to tap into the peaceful feeling anytime she chose. She was amazed at how quickly she was able to change her focus, relax and maintain her equilibrium in the middle of the situation using this simple breathing technique.

It takes consistent practice to maintain tension in your body and it will take consistent practice to undo it. The following technique will help you better to let go of that tension.

RELAXATION EXERCISE:

Relax stretched out on a bed; take three deep breaths. Begin to relax all the muscles in the feet, allow them to go loose and limp, completely and totally relaxed, completely and totally relaxed. Now the calf muscles, let them go loose and limp, completely and totally relaxed, completely and totally relaxed. Now the pelvic area, the buttocks muscles, let them go loose and limp, completely and totally relaxed, completely and totally relaxed. Now the stomach area, all the internal organs, let them go loose and limp, completely relaxed – take a deep breath and let them relax even more. Now the chest muscles and the back muscles, let them go loose and limp, completely and totally relaxed, completely and totally relaxed. Now the arms and the hands, let them go loose and limp, completely and totally relaxed, completely relaxed. Now the shoulder and neck muscles, let them go loose and limp, completely and totally relaxed, completely and totally relaxed. Now even the scalp, let all the tension flow out of the scalp, let it go loose and limp, completely and totally relaxed, completely and totally relaxed. Now the forehead and the muscles around the eyes, let them

71

go loose and limp, completely and totally relaxed, completely and totally relaxed. Let your jaw drop slightly and let the cheek muscles go loose and limp, completely and totally relaxed, completely and totally relaxed. Visualize yourself on a soft white cloud, surrounded by blue sky, completely and totally relaxed. Take a deep breath and feel your whole body completely and totally relaxed. You are filled with a feeling of peace and serenity. You are beginning to be aware of your body again as you slowly bring your attention back to the room, bringing back with you that peaceful relaxed feeling.

This relaxation technique should be practiced every day. Focusing on relaxing the individual muscles helps to keep your mind in the present. With each practice session you will find it easier to reach a deeper state of relaxation.

LEARNING TO CONCENTRATE:

Before you can begin to mediate, the mind must be brought under control. Learning how to concentrate, to focus, means being able to quiet the constant chatter that goes on in your head.

It has been shown in studies of successful people, that one of the traits they share is the ability to clearly focus on any goal they set. Following is a technique that if practiced consistently will help you control the direction of your mind and your life.

CONCENTRATION TECHNIQUE:

Sitting in a chair with eyes closed, visualize a movie screen in your mind with a large wall clock on it, like a schoolroom clock. Mentally begin to follow the second hand around the clock as it moves from one to twelve. Repeat this three times. If your mind wanders, don't get upset; just gently bring it back to the clock. After three circles, take a deep breath and rest. Practice this technique as many times a day as convenient. The more you practice the easier it will become.

Another method is to lie on a bed and pick out a point or a spot on the ceiling and hold your attention at that point. If the mind wanders, gently bring it back to the point of focus. With persistence it will become easier to control and to hold your thoughts where you want them.

Any object can be used to practice your concentration. Some people use a candle flame, an apple, even a leaf on a tree; the aim is to begin controlling the unruly mind.

DEEP BREATHING

Correct breathing is the cornerstone of any of the techniques practiced. Deep, diaphragmatic breathing will automatically relax every muscle in your body. Done correctly, it is impossible to remain tense. If for no other reason, learning deep breathing can help to relieve everyday stress.

DEEP BREATHING EXERCISE

Stretch out on your back, arms resting easily by your side. Slowly breathe in through the nose, mentally observing the breath flowing first to the stomach area. The stomach should rise (like a balloon) as it fills with air; hold the breath for a moment, then take more air into the upper chest. Hold the breath for a moment and then slowly expel the air through the mouth, allowing air to be pushed out from the stomach area first (like squeezing a tube of toothpaste from the bottom). The stomach will fall and then the chest gently falls. It will feel almost like the rolling of a wave with the stomach rising, the chest rising, the stomach falling and then the chest falling. When done correctly, it relaxes every muscle in the body. It is automatic, the muscles must relax.

There are a number of benefits derived from deep breathing. When you hold the breath, it saturates the red blood cells with oxygen. The oxygen helps to cleanse the toxins from the system. It helps to get oxygen to the brain to promote clearer thinking, and is a wonderful tool to use in stressful situations.

The best time to practice this exercise is just before going to sleep at night. Begin by taking three deep breaths, getting the feel of the rhythm while continuing to let go. If you try too many series of breaths, you may experience tingling in your hands and feet or get lightheaded. It is best to stop and rest until you get used to the increased oxygen in your system.

74

SCRAMBLING: (Tony Robbins, 1992)

In Tony Robbins book, <u>Awaken the Giant Within</u>, he recommends a method he calls Scrambling. The idea is to change the negative images we hold in our mind into comical situations. By scrambling these images we can make them less forbidding and eventually change our inner perception.

SCRAMBLING TECHNIQUE:

"A SIMPLE WAY OF BREAKING A PATTERN IS BY SCRAMBLING THE SENSATIONS WE LINK TO OUR MEMORIES. For example: if your boss yells at you and you mentally rerun that experience the rest of the day, picturing him or her yelling at you over and over again, then you'll feel progressively worse. Why not just take this record in your mind and scratch it so many times that you can't experience those feelings anymore? Maybe you can even make it funny.

"The scramble pattern: 1) See the situation in your mind that was bothering you so much. Picture it as a movie. Don't feel upset about it; just watch it one time, seeing everything that happened. 2) Take the same experience and turn it into a cartoon: If somebody said something, watch them swallow their words! Run the movie in reverse, change the colors of the images so that everybody's faces are rainbow-colored. If there's someone in particular who upsets you, cause their ears to grow very large like Mickey Mouse's, and their nose grow like Pinocchio. Do this at least a dozen times back and forth, sideways, scratching the record of your imagery. With tremendous speed and humor link weird sounds to the old image ... this will definitely change the sensations. The key to this whole process is the speed and level of humor and exaggeration you can link to it.

Why does it work? Because all of our feelings are based on the images we focus on in our minds and the sounds and sensations we link to those specific images." (Tony Robbins). One way of breaking the pattern is to just stop doing it.

STOPPING UNWANTED THOUGHTS:

Stopping unwanted thoughts is another technique offered by Davis, McKay, and Eshelman/Relaxation and Stress Reduction Workbook.

"Stopping unwanted thoughts takes consistent motivation. Select a thought you want to extinguish; close your eyes and imagine a stressful situation. Interrupt the unwanted thought with a startling interruption such as a bell ringing (timer) or shout stop, or stand up quickly and walk around. Think of what will work for you to redirect your mind to something less destructive and more constructive."

What are some of the questions you can ask yourself to stop unwanted thoughts?

1. Who is in control here?

2. Do I want to give someone that much power over me?

3. Am I a helpless puppet?

4. What do I want?

5. How do I feel?

6. Is the situation worth the pain?

An example: In a relationship situation, Diane spent days replaying an emotional scene that caused constant stress and pain. After two days of creating scenarios and imagining all kinds of retorts, she realized how much this individual was controlling her life. Exhausted and bored with the unending ritual, Diane made a decision never to let this individual disrupt her life again. The feeling behind her decision was so strong that there was an immediate emotional release and she was able to stop the cycle of distress.

SELF-TALK

How do you talk to yourself? When you become aware of your thoughts, you will probably find a running dialogue of negative judgements; statements such as, "I should be doing this, or I shouldn't be doing that." Statements that tend to diminish your self-esteem.

Albert Ellis in his book, A Guide to Rational Living, states that the mind is often filled with irrational thoughts and beliefs about life based strictly on emotions. He believes that emotions have nothing to do with actual events. Your mind colors everything you see and hear through the filter of your own experience. Your perception of what is happening may have nothing to do with reality. Your self-talk filters your perception and determines how you respond to the situation. That is why two people can be experiencing the same event, yet come away with two totally different impressions.

You might be sitting on a mountaintop as you watch a beautiful sunset against the backdrop of a lush forest. But you are unaware of its beauty because the thoughts in your head are making you sad because you don't have someone to share it with. While another person can be ecstatic to be alone on that same hilltop and breathless with the beauty of the sunset. The scene is the same; the perception (emotion) is different. What you say inwardly to yourself will create your response to life.

If your self-talk is constantly putting you down with statements such as:

I'm not very smart.

Why do I always do things wrong?

No one likes me anyway.

It will create feelings of anxiety, anger, rage, guilt, and a sense of worthlessness. Your body will react to negative self-talk by producing tension, toxins, and stress.

"At the root of all irrational thinking is the assumption that things are done to you." (Davis, McKay, Eshelman/The Relaxation and Stress Reduction Workbook). For example: When a friend 'makes' you angry by always being late, you take it personally, when in reality, the friend is always late for everything. To keep from getting angry you can change your perception (you won't change him/her), and gauge your time accordingly. Allow for his late arrival by asking him to be there earlier, hoping he will then be on time. Tell him that you must leave by a certain time and if he is not there within 15 minutes, you will have to leave without him ... and then do it. He will probably be angry with you for not playing his game, but at least you will not be angry.

How you see a situation and the self-talk you indulge in will determine how you respond. If your self-talk is angry and negative, you will respond by becoming angry and negative.

Be aware of the statements and questions you make to yourself on a daily basis. They become the building blocks of your future. Replace negative self-talk with positive phrases that support and increase your self-esteem.

Your own thoughts, you own self-talk can be your best friend or your worst enemy.

MEDITATION

It is difficult to describe meditation. Meditation is an experience. There are three steps to consider. The first step is learning how to concentrate. The second step is meditation. Third step is contemplation. To meditate successfully, you must first learn to control your mind. The chatter n the mind is controlled by concentrating on an object, a word, a mantra, or a sound. It acts as a focus to keep you centered and quiet.

Meditation is not prayer in the normal sense. In meditation you are listening rather than talking. An example would be: you are home alone and have just turned out the lights to go to bed. You know there is no one else there, but all of a sudden you hear a noise and you are totally focused trying to hear it again … listening.

Also, it is like being in the eye of a storm; the center is very quiet, you are aware of things going on around you, but you are focused in the quiet center, not disturbed by the outer noise. It is similar to being so intensely interested in a good book that you could be in the midst of a crowd and still be so absorbed that you do not hear what is being said.

Meditation helps to quiet the chatter in the mind so the body can rest to help heal the body from the damages of stress.

MEDITATION TECHNIQUE #1

Sit erect in a straight back chair. Take three deep breaths and relax. Slowly imagine your energy flowing in through your fingertips, up through your arms, feeling it as warmth as it flows to your Solar Plexus (just below the sternum). Hold your attention there briefly, feeling that warmth. Again, draw your energy up through your feet and legs letting it flow to the solar plexus and hold your attention there briefly. Begin repeating the word "peace" over and over. If your mind wanders, don't get upset; gently bring your attention back to the word. Meditate for about ten minutes in the beginning or less according to your time limit. When you have completed your meditation, gently bring your attention back to the body and back to the room; don't hurry. Bring back that feeling of peace and harmony with you.

MEDITATION TECHNIQUE #2

As you sit erect in a straight back chair, let your arms rest at your side with the hands palm up in your lap, feet flat on the floor. Mentally check your body for tension, the neck, the shoulders, arms, hands, chest, legs? As you take a deep breath, focus on the area where you have any tension and mentally tell those muscles to relax. After you let go of the tension, focus on your breathing. Watch it flow in and out at the tip of your nose. Feel as though the breath is filling the inside of your head and then flowing out as you exhale. It sometimes helps to imagine the breath as a light or feel it as warmth. Gently watch the breath for approximately four breaths. Now taking another deep breath, rest for a moment with the sense that you don't need to do anything, just rest.

When you have completed your meditation, slowly bring your attention back to your body and the room.

To be effective, a technique must be practiced every day until it becomes an automatic response. The person who can control his thoughts can control his anger and will have more control over a situation than the one lost in his emotions.

In summary, you are attempting to gain more control over your life. It will take a mental shift as well as a physical shift to make the changes you desire.

MENTAL SHIFT:

- Learn to relax

- Learn to focus your thoughts

- Learn to meditate

PHYSICAL SHIFT:

- Learn new behaviors

- Reinforce the new behaviors

- Attend workshops

- Join a support group

A statistical study to measure relapse behavior, conducted by researcher Nancy Mann, showed that in order to maintain change it was important to: 1) consciously choose new behaviors to replace the old one; 2) reinforce these new behaviors with repetition and emotional intensity; and 3) seek or create a network of support from family and friends. The study showed that support from loved ones is an important link to long term success.

CHAPTER TEN

SETTING GOALS

CREATING YOUR FUTURE

> **A Goal must be:**
>
> **POSITIVE**
>
> **SPECIFIC &**
>
> **MEASURABLE."**

With your values and beliefs clarified, you are ready to make new choices and set new goals.

A goal is something positive that you *will* to be done. The act of organizing your thoughts and ideas and writing them down reinforces those thoughts and ideas. You may not achieve them all, but you will find yourself accomplishing more and more with the practice of goal setting.

Goals are simply changes you want to make in your life. They can be large (going to medical school) or small (writing a letter to a friend). External (I'd like to double my salary in five years) or internal (I'd like to feel better about myself).

A goal must be specific, positive result you wish to achieve. It must be measurable. Stating that happiness is your goal is not specific enough. How do you measure happiness? What does it mean to you? If your goal is financial security, what does that look like? $50,000 a year salary. $100,000 in the bank, a nest egg for retirement? A goal must be specific in order to achieve it. In the beginning setting your goals may seem like a monumental task. Listing them by priority can simplify them and allow you to deal with each step – one at a time.

Realistic approach: Set simple, easily reachable goals in some areas and tougher, longer-term goals in others ... always keeping sight of the overall quality of your life.

The formula:

$50,000 income + $50,000 pension fund + $50,000 savings

= FINANCIAL SECURITY

To define a goal you must:

1. Be specific

2. State a desired result

3. Set dates and dollars (when appropriate)

4. Make goals positive

5. State what you *want*, not what you *don't* want.

If earning $50,000 a year salary is your goal, what are you doing to reach it? If you are making $30,000 a year now, what will it take to reach your goal? Ask yourself...

1. Am I happy in the work I am now doing?

2. Will this job allow me to make $50,000 a year?

3. Do I need more experience and training? How can I get that training? Don't wait for someone else to arrange it for you. Decide what training you will need and go after it. Design your own training program. This is what Susan did:

When Susan's talent appraisal came due, she sat down with her boss and discussed her goals and what her aspirations were within the company. She told him she would like to be promoted to account executive but knew she needed more specific training.

Susan suggested that she design a training program and submit it to him for his approval. Her boss readily agreed since it freed up his time.

In the following year, when it came time for Susan's raise, she reminded her boss of her request for a promotion. It was obvious with his busy schedule he had forgotten, but was more than happy to consider it if she would send him a memo on the projects and responsibilities she had been handling.

Susan promptly sat down and described her duties, also attached a copy of the completed training.

She received the title and the raise.

4. Do you need to go back to school for more education? If you moan at the prospect, realize you must be willing to do what it takes to get where you want to go. Mary was willing:

At 38, divorced after 18 years of marriage and raising five children, she decided to go back to work. After 18 years of not working, she was overwhelmed with the prospect.

In spite of her fears, she found an Executive Secretary's job with a manager who had confidence in her ability to learn. After two years in the business world, she decided to go back to college and was able to receive four full years of scholarships and graduated with an Associate degree as well as a Bachelor's degree in Science. There were momentous decisions along the way, but with her willingness to take the risk and with support of her family and friends she was able to achieve her goal.

5. Educational assistance is often offered in some firms to enhance job skills.

6. Realistically, how long will it take you to achieve your goal? Set a date – this is important because it makes your commitment more concrete. Look at all the ways you *can* do it, not why you *can't* do it.

As doubts and fears emerge, recognize that you have them, but don't let them stop you. You may feel you don't have the skills or knowledge, but with persistence and determination they can be acquired.

Write out your goals clearly and take the steps necessary to accomplish it. Again, don't wait for the perfect moment or someone else to do it for you.

TAKE ACTION!

The next step in your formula is your retirement program. What information do you need to make a decision?

1. Does your company have a policy?

2. Are you covered sufficiently?

3. Do you need more insurance?

4. What other options do you have to increase your retirement benefits?

IMPORTANT NOTE:

Before you make any decision, make sure you have all the information you need. Do your homework. Find out what is out there for you to draw on before you start deciding it is impossible.

Make a list of the steps you need to take to gather your information. Make appointments with the individuals who can give you this information. Set dates and times to meet with them, thereby making a commitment to yourself to get it done.

If you are not already in a savings program, set up an appointment with a financial counselor and go over different ways that you can save that perhaps you had not considered. Get books on finance from the library; talk with friends to get ideas. Again, set dates and times to do this. Be willing to do what it takes to achieve your goal.

What other resources do you have? Can you give up a few luxuries – or better yet – look at ways you have been spending money. It has a way of falling through the cracks. Do you have talents you are not using? A business woman in a busy advertising agency teaches one night a week at a local community college in the continuing education program – a position that not only brings her extra cash, but is something she thoroughly enjoys. The extra work does not have to be a punishment. On the contrary, it can and should be something you enjoy doing. You are after all creating a happier lifestyle for yourself. Be creative with alternatives.

In the process of your goal setting – if you get stuck making a decision, use the Field Force Analysis technique mentioned in Chapter [9]. List all the pros and cons relating to the goal or decision. If you have more negative responses than positive, be cautious about a "yes" decision.

One of the fascinating things about goals is that, as you set out in the direction of one goal, new ideas and opportunities begin to open up, which without the seeking, would not have been available to you.

Buckminster Fuller, a noted scientist, explains that there is a natural rhythm or energy that is set in motion when you start out on the path toward a goal. As you begin searching, meeting new people, asking questions, information is opened to you that literally expands your vision of possibilities. You may find yourself setting new and loftier goals as a result of the information you gather along the way. Failure to reach your original goal is not failure if it motivated you to search and question and ultimately reach an even higher goal.

At this point you may find yourself having problems deciding what your goals are. Ask yourself – what do I want from life? Following is an exercise that can help you clarify what you do want:

Find a spot where you can sit quietly. It would be helpful to have a friend or spouse prompt you with the questions, but you can also do it alone.

Close your eyes and imagine your mind as a blank movie screen. Now write, produce and direct your own mini-movie about your ideal future. If you can see it clearly and can get into the feeling of it, you *can* make it happen.

Ask yourself the following questions:

- If you could have it your way, what would your life be like? Create a mental picture.

- Would you have a family?

- Live alone?

- Live in a big house?

- Live in a small house?

- Describe your house in detail.

- Would you work or stay at home?

- Would you be a business man/woman?

- Would you own your own business?

- What kind of person would you like to be?

- Describe this person:

  - ✓ Gentle

  - ✓ Kind

  - ✓ Strong

  - ✓ Independent

  - ✓ Serene

  - ✓ Exciting

  - ✓ Bold

  - ✓ Aggressive

- What kind of atmosphere would you surround yourself with?

BUSINESS LIFE:

What kind of work would you like to do?

- Working with your hands?

- Working with people?

- Counseling?

- Writing?

- Acting?

- Selling?

- Business management?

> What kind of business would you like to manage?

✓ Describe the people you would work with.

✓ Describe your office.

✓ What income would you like to make?

- What do you enjoy dong for fun?

Of course you can add as many questions as you like, but this will give you an idea of how to go about doing it.

Visualize what you want as if it already exists. In this process, don't try to analyze or solve anything. Don't begin arguing with yourself about why it can't be done. Just pretend that all the elements are there for you to achieve your goal. Before change becomes a reality you have to believe it is possible. All great inventions began first as one man's dream or vision.

When you have completed your own personal movie, take the time to write it down. Draw a picture in words underlining the important elements. Writing solidifies and reinforces your thoughts and ideas.

List each desire or goal, such as the new house, the new job, the new behavior, etc. As you list each item, ask yourself, am I willing to do what it takes to make this happen? Do I really want this? If you had it, would you take it? If the answer -- coming from the *feeling* level -- is no, then don't waste your time. Focus your energy on the things that are important to you.

Again, to achieve your goals you must be:

1.   CLEAR ABOUT WHAT YOU WANT.

2.   ABLE TO VISUALIZE IT.

3.   WILLING TO ACT ON IT.

Alice acted on her desire. She was a school teacher working with handicapped children in a Georgia school system. For years she had been talking about taking a trip to Europe. But it was always with the attitude of "but of course, I can't because..." I finally asked her, "Do you really want to go? ... Yes ... then tell me all the reasons you *can* go."

Working together, we discussed all the steps necessary for her to be able to go to Europe.

First, she *accepted* the *possibility* of going to Europe. Second, she made a commitment to go. Third, she took action.

Her first act was to design a strategy. She gathered all the information she would need to plan.

- When she wanted to go (dates)

- Tours available and costs

- Passport papers

- Wardrobe

Although Alice didn't know where the money would come from, she began making her plans. She believed it was possible and was willing to put the energy behind it to *make* it happen.

Here are some of the things she did:

1. Opened a special vacation savings account.

2. Sold many of her unneeded items at flea markets.

3. Signed up for market research projects, which paid her $25 each time, she participated.

4. Discovered money in her savings account she had forgotten. Her grandmother had left her $1,000 in her will and Alice had put it in her savings for an emergency and promptly forgotten about it.

5. Although she didn't have a credit record, she

was able to borrow the final $1,000 from a bank on her personal signature.

6. Alice was able to sublet her apartment for the seven weeks she was away in Europe.

After an exciting whirlwind tour of Europe, Alice is now planning a trip to the Orient.

Alice had to believe it was possible before she could see the resources she had at hand.

If you are not willing to look at alternatives and be persistent, then you probably don't want it badly enough. Ask yourself – have you failed to accomplish something because you *can't* do it, or is it because you *won't* do it?

WHY WE FAIL TO ACHIEVE OUR GOALS:

Every choice you make is based on your:

1. Past experience

2. Your beliefs and expectations

3. Your values

4. Your inner thoughts/self-talk

5. Your feelings

All of the above will influence the decisions you make. Your mind will pull from your experience, your values, and your feelings to either encourage or discourage you to take action.

To achieve the goals you have set, your goals must be in alignment with your value system. You cannot expect new results based on old ideas.

To achieve any goal a person must "act."

1. Examine and develop values (make sure values aren't in conflict).

2. Define the goal or solution.

3. Develop alternatives

4. Decide which course of action is best.

<u>MAJOR LIFE AREAS</u>

1. *Self-esteem.* Ex.: I'll write down three different things I like about myself every day for a week.

2. *Health and Fitness*: Ex: I'm going to cut back to one cup of coffee per day ... starting?

3. *Communication*: I'm gong to take a workshop in assertiveness training to help me learn to say no. Date: ____.

4. *Relationships*: Ex: I'll initiate a talk with my partner about where our relationship is headed on ____.

5. *Career/Lifework*: Ex: I'm going to look into job training programs that can help me upgrade my job skills. Date ____.

6. *Finances/Personal Wealth*: Ex: For one month, I will write down everything I buy so I'll know where my money goes.

7. *Life Crisis*: Ex: I'll find out about support groups for people with my health problems ... or I'll read a book about coping with grief.

8. *Your Spiritual Self*: Ex: I'm going to buy a book on meditation or each day for the next two weeks, I'm going to take a walk in the woods.

PERSONAL DEVELOPMENT GOALS

A. List your goals for personal development:

1. Next to each of these goals, write down the time frame you plan to accomplish them i.e., within 1, 3, 5, 10, 20 years.

2. Select your top three personal development goals and under each one, write a paragraph describing why you're committed to achieving this goal.

B. List your "Things" goals -- Same as 1. and 2. above.

C. List your "Economic" goals – Same as 1. and 2. above.

D. For each of your top nine goals, write down one action you can take right away to begin progress toward achieving it.

 1. Take that action today!

 2. Do the Rocking chair test to help you commit to accomplishing each of your goals:

    Imagine yourself much older, sitting in your rocking chair and looking back on your life. First, as if you had not achieved your goals; then what it would be like if you had achieved them. (Experience the pain that would follow not doing it along with the pleasure that would come from having reached your goals.)

Goal setting is not a win or lose situation. It is a way of gaining control over your life on a day to day basis.

- Don't try to set goals for other people. If they don't achieve it, you'll feel resentful or even responsible for their failure.

- Set short range expectations for your goals:

    I will "never" eat ice cream again ... too overwhelming.

    I will not eat ice cream today!

- There is a tendency to give up on long range goals because it is harder to see progress on a day-to-day basis.

- Goals must be a real challenge and be big enough to create the excitement necessary for accomplishment. Big but not unrealistic.

ACTION PHASE:

Develop programs of activity to reach desired goals. Develop a series of steps. "Where I am to where I want to be ..."

MAKING CHOICES:

Life is all about making choices. The choices you make will lead to success or failure. These choices are based on life experiences, values, beliefs, and emotions. Rather than basing your choices on a limited set of guidelines and rules, begin to expand your vision by combining reason, (the Left New Brain), creativity (the Right New Brain) and feeling (the Visceral Brain) to create an Wholistic/Balanced lifestyle.

THE WHOLISITC BRAIN:

When the Old Brain and the New Brain work as a unit they bring together the strengths of the emotional, the rational, and the creative parts of the brain to create what we call the Wholistic Brain. This balance lifts man above his basic animal instincts and gives him the power to rationally think things through before acting impulsively.

If you continually allow impulse to rule your life, without the balance of the rational and creative sides of the brain, you will continue to be frustrated by failure. By being more aware of the choices you make and why you are making them, you can better control the direction of your life. The choices you make will reflect in the world around you. So choose wisely.

Theresa Williams Firster

Theresa Firster has a degree in Mental Health and has done extensive work as a group leader and instructor for: Columbus Georgia Police Department as a DUI instructor, led courses in stress reduction and attitude assessment for a division of Hew; was an adjunct professor and consultant at Columbus College relating to stress and time management; instructed a course at Oglethorpe University in Atlanta on the Brain & Stress; guest instructor on stress management for Emory University Employees, Atlanta Ga. She is currently working as a consultant in Human Resources.

Dr. Waino Suojanen

Dr. Waino Suojanen is a retired Professor of Management at Georgia State University's College of Business Administration, where he specialized in addictive behaviors and stress-related disease. He publishes and lectures extensively in the United States and abroad on his integrative approach to behavior management. He has also served as the Director for the R&D Management Program at Eglin Air Force Base, and is currently a consultant to the Management Training Agency of the U.S. Army and to Xerox Corporation. Dr. Suojanen received his B.S. from the University of Vermont, his MBA from Harvard University and his Ph.D. from the University of California at Berkeley. He is the author of the Brain and Stress, published by Georgia State University Press in 1983 and The Dynamics of Management which won the McKinsey Foundation Award in 1966.